The Adventures of Mighty Milo

Godly parents – Milo chooses his family

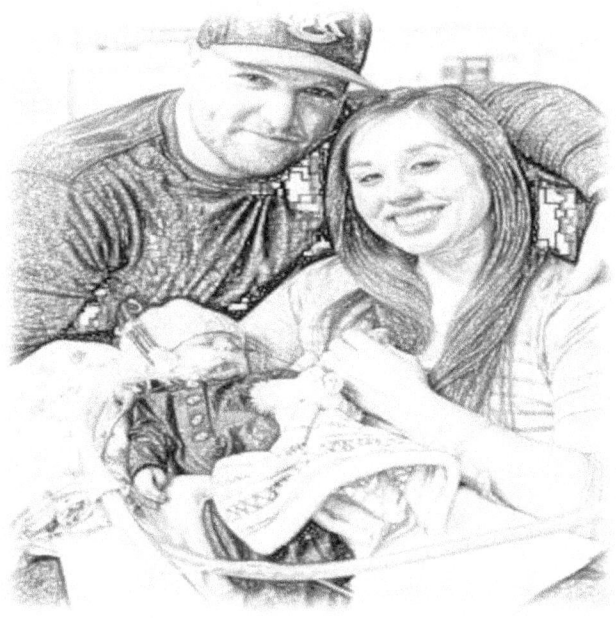

Written in collaboration with

Milo Dallen Myers & Nana Barby

The book was written as a birthday gift to my daughter Shelly Myers. I had no idea what to give her for her birthday the year after she lost Milo until the light bulb went off in my head. "Write a book" my mind said and I replied, "yes I will from Milo's perspective on why he chose his parents".

This was the inspiration from above to offer comfort and love to my beautiful and caring daughter, Michelle Myers.

With love always,

Mom

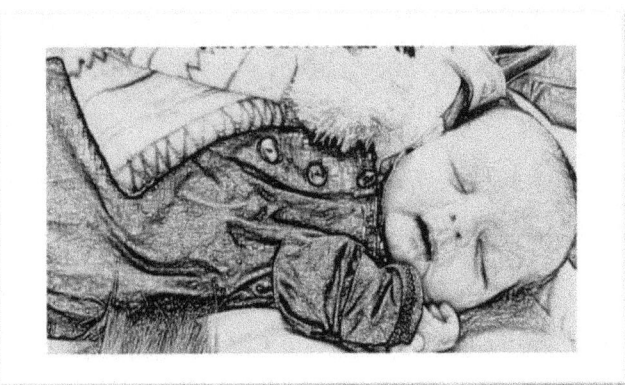

Hi, my name is Milo Dallin Myers. They call me Mighty because my journey here to earth to meet my parents and struggle to remain was difficult. And I was a warrior and did my very best when I arrived. But it wasn't easy for mommy & daddy, not from the very beginning.

You see, my mommy and daddy tried for several years to have a baby and then found out they couldn't the normal way. So they entered a contest through 97.1 ZHT in Salt Lake City, Utah called "Win a Baby Contest". And yes, they won! Out of 40 contestants, they won. Miracle of miracles!

I'm an IVF baby and it truly is a miracle that I was born. Even more of a miracle that I lived 19 days because I was born with CDH, Congenital Diaphragmatic Hernia.

Because I have Godly, amazing and sweet parents that I chose, the journey to Earth, in my mommy's tummy and being born was worth it! Here is my story.

Let's start at the beginning so you can truly appreciate my journey and my loving parents, Jason and Shelly Myers.

Jason and Shelly were married in the Draper, Utah Temple on May 18, 2013. They met because of my Nana Barby when she lived in Oklahoma, but that's another amazing love story.

I was born on August 4, 2019 and the labor and delivery was long and difficult. My mommy Shelly went to the hospital with breathing difficulties due to the fluid buildup caused by CDH. My daddy, Jason, drove me and mommy to Utah Primary Children's Hospital from Orem to Salt Lake praying they would get there in time to help my mommy's breathing.

When they arrived, mommy and I were rushed into the labor and delivery room in the hospital, and it was quite nice. Daddy was by our side the entire time even when he was so exhausted from lack of sleep. My mommy was in labor for a really long time and at one point went into Pasmo (reverse labor). You see, I really wasn't ready to come out into the world yet. It was warm and safe inside of my mommy and I felt happy in there with her.

I chose my parents to be my family when I was above, before I came into the world. I watched them as they struggled to get pregnant with two failed IVF attempts and their grace, elegance and persistence made me want to be their son. I watched them every day from above in my spiritual realm. Each day they loved each other and each night they prayed together, read scriptures and my daddy always kissed my mommy on the forehead. Kind of like the picture below. I just knew they would love me and do all they could for me, even if I wasn't going to stay very long.

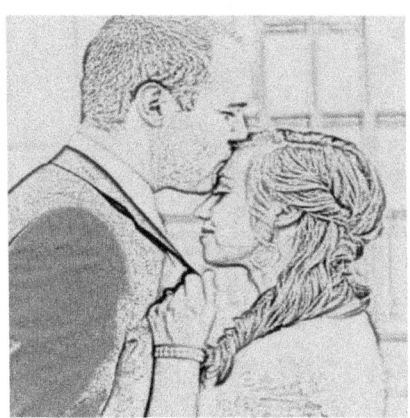

IVF – Invitro Fertilization is laborious and daily injections of hormones and other things clearly showed me that Shelly and Jason really wanted to be parents, my parents.

Shelly told Nana Barby, my grandma, the good news on December 7th, 2018 at 3:30 p.m. She cried with tears and said was "pregnant" with me. Nana was so happy because she wanted me to be with her daughter Shelly, with all her heart. So her prayers to Heavenly Father were answered along with my mommy and daddy's. Many people in the family and even friends of my parents were praying, and it was beautiful to see all the support they were getting and would get in the future.

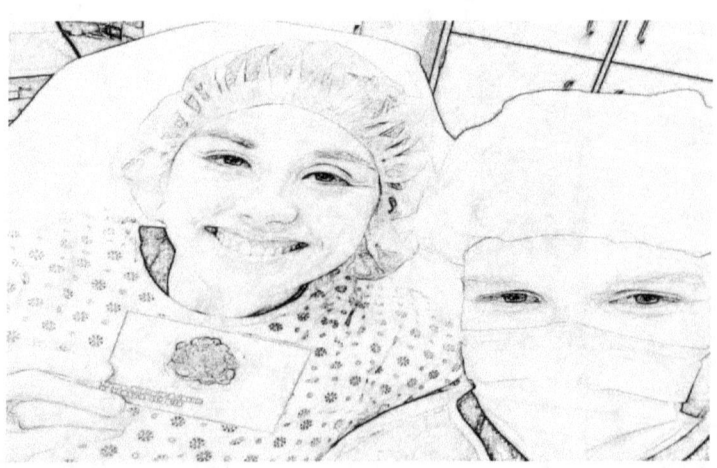

Mommy was a trooper and exercised to stay healthy while daddy cooked all the meals for me and mommy. It was so comforting to hear mommy's voice and daddies too! Around the second trimester during one of the tests, the doctors told my parents there were some issues and concerns. They noticed what appeared to be CDH, Congenital Diaphragmatic Hernia but didn't know the level of severity and wouldn't know until I was born. Devastating news to my parents but they vowed to have me and keep moving forward regardless of the outcome. They loved me!

There were many challenges and difficulties during the remaining pregnancy, and even through all of that, my parents loved me. There was one time that mommy was getting a test, and I was sleeping really well. The technician told mommy that if I didn't wake up and move around that she would have to go upstairs for several hours of testing. Just then mommy spoke to me and said I needed to wake up and move around, and being a good little boy, I did. Just goes to prove that I heard everything she said to me, and I followed her wishes. Well, I kept growing inside of mommy's belly and soon she looked very pregnant indeed.

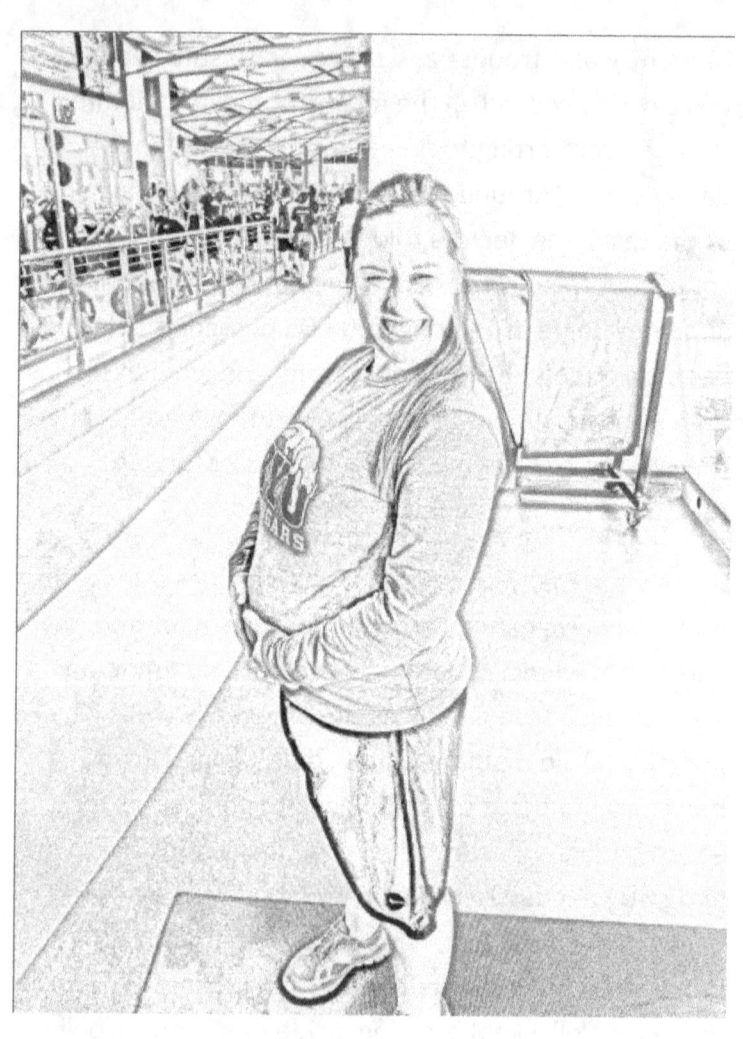

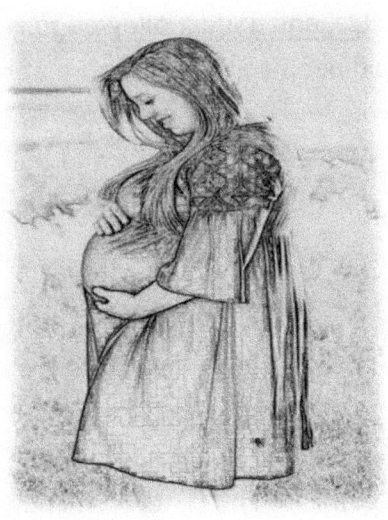

The days and months passed ever so quickly and the countdown to my arrival was coming soon. When August arrived, it gave way to new concerns and new doctors involved in my care upon my birth. Mommy and I tried to have a natural birth but when she went into Pasmo, I stopped right where I was. I didn't like to be moved or turned, and I really just wanted to stay inside with mommy. Soon the decision was made to perform a C-section to bring me into the world. Mommy was tough as nails and daddy was right by our side the entire time. When I came out, I was a healthy weight and size, 7 pounds and 19 inches long but I was blue, and my breathing was very shallow. They rushed me into the NICU, and daddy followed to keep an eye on me. He told people at my funeral that he was torn between his wife and his son, but mommy told him to come be with me. See how loving and thoughtful she is? Always thinking of others, not herself. I sure do love her!

Well, daddy was crying and pleading with Heavenly Father to keep me here on Earth while the nurses and doctors were busy trying to help me breathe. The doctor told my dad that I wouldn't last long if my oxygen didn't come up and that just made daddy even more sad. But then, suddenly, in comes mommy being wheeled in her hospital bed by the nursing staff. She placed her hand on me and our spirits connected instantly. My breathing got better, and my oxygen increased because mommy and daddy were there, loving me.

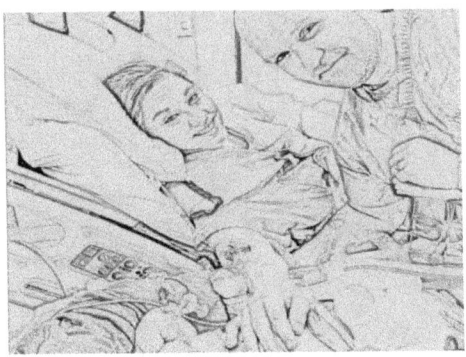

My struggles weren't over though. I was placed on the ECMO machine because my one lung was too small and the other needed help. Extracorporeal membrane oxygenation (ECMO) is a treatment that uses a pump to circulate blood through an artificial lung back into the bloodstream of a very ill baby.

You see CDH causes the organs in your abdomen, like the liver, intestines, stomach and such to go into your chest because the diaphragm, which is a muscle that helps you breathe and keeps the organs separated from one another. Like the lungs and heart are on the top and your stomach, liver, intestines and such are on the bottom. When you have CDH the diaphragm muscle doesn't close, and your organs slip up into your chest.

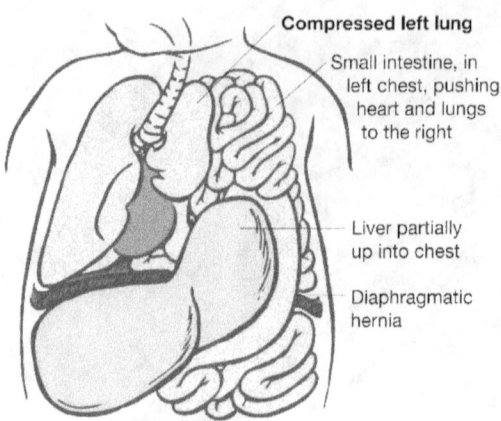

Mine was pretty bad and my lungs and heart were on the right side of my chest.   So, the ECMO machine was working on my behalf.

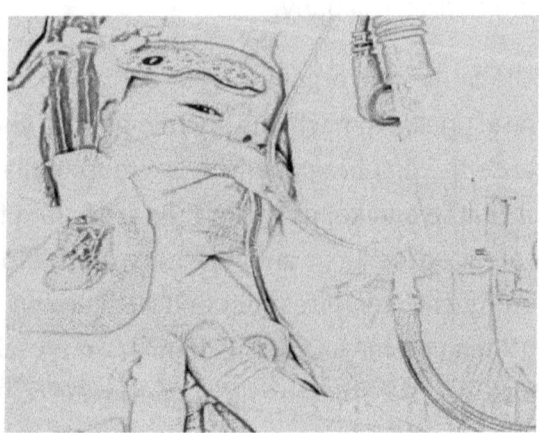

The doctors decided to move my organs down to my abdomen with surgery while I was on ECMO because I wasn't stable enough to breathe on my own without it. I was a medical first because I was the first baby to have surgery while still on ECMO. Medical history made on behalf **of Mighty Milo Myers**. I want you to know that I didn't suffer because mommy and daddy and all the nurses and doctors made sure I was given medicine so I wouldn't feel pain.

I felt pretty good after my surgery, and it looked like I was going to be alright. Until the doctors came in to talk to mommy and daddy again. Now there were issues with my small heart, my kidneys and other internal things and that just wasn't good to hear.

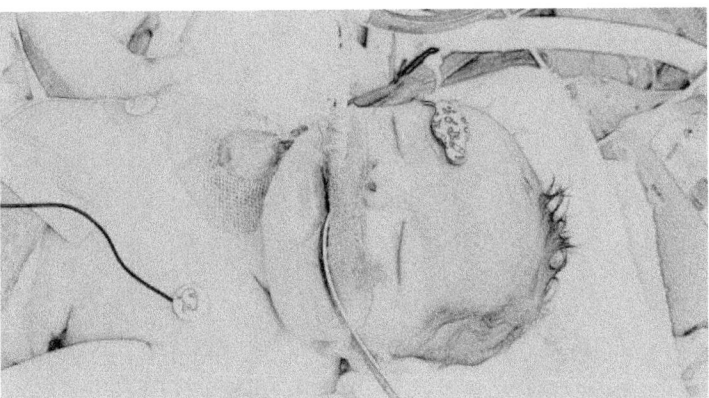

Overwhelmed by all of this, mommy and daddy reached out to family and said to come meet me because the future was uncertain. My grandma and grandpa Orr were first to meet me and then grandma and grandpa Harmon.

I had aunts and uncles who came to visit me too! My Nana Barby was last to meet me, and she stayed for several days. She read stories to me and cheered me on through my procedure telling me how special I was and that I could do anything.

It was wonderful to have my family, all of them, come see me while I was here on Earth. I picked a great family to be my own! And my parents? Well, they are the best ever! They loved and cherished me the entire 9 months I was growing and the 19 days I lived on Earth with them. It was a beautiful time, and I was loved by so many of the clinical team that came to see me and my parents every day.

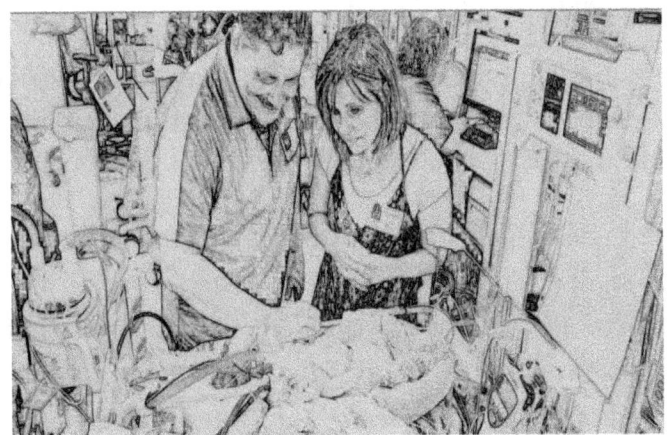

I wish my story had a happy ending, but my life was filled with purpose and meaning. I brought people all over the world together for one purpose, praying for me and my medical issues. People who didn't even believe in God were praying for me.

I put up a fight fit for a warrior, God's Heavenly Warrior. The greatest part of my short life on Earth was spending all those days with my parents, Jason and Shelly.

I felt their love, them holding my hand, reading me stories, daddy reading me scriptures and mommy smiling with loving encouragement. I spent the last of my ten hours with mommy & daddy. It was wonderful! We sat together like the family we are, a real family! And I felt their enduring love, even now I feel them in Heaven above.

I want you to know mommy and daddy that I'm watching over you. And I'll be with you soon, I promise. I'm so happy I chose you to be my family and grateful that we spent that time together in the NICU. But mostly I'm grateful that you loved me. You loved me throughout the entire journey from beginning to the very last part.

I LOVE YOU!   Your son Milo 🤍

The following pages are stories about my journey, letters from my mommy and pictures in this book.

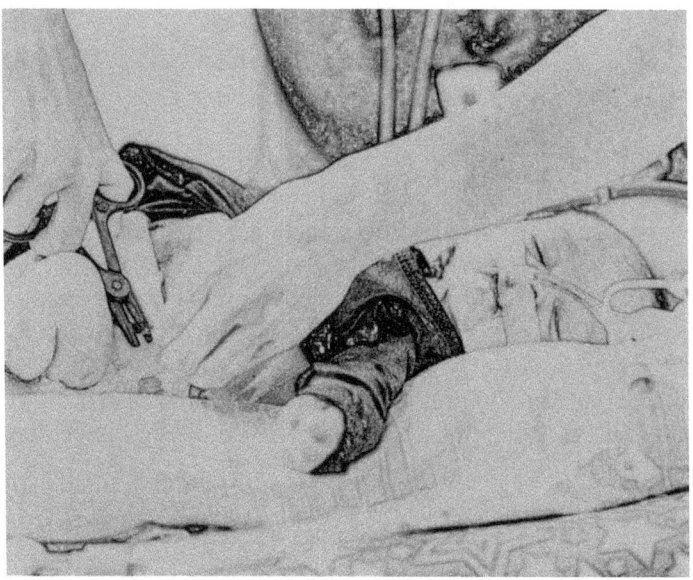

Mighty Milo

This is my story as told by my one of my NICU nurses, Angie Birkeland, at my funeral.

MIGHTY MILO MYERS

Hello everyone, my name is Angie Birkeland and I was one of the lucky nurses that got to care for Milo during his NICU stay.

First, I want to tell Jason and Shelly how honored I am to have been asked to speak tonight about Milo and his journey. When Shelly texted me to ask if I would speak, I asked her how long they wanted me to talk. I got an immediate response back saying, "Jason would like you to take a full hour with an accompanying PowerPoint in Times New Roman". I'm kind of disappointed that I don't have a PowerPoint prepared Jason, but I did type this up in Times New Roman. I hope that is sufficient.

Tonight, my goal is to share Milo's story, his life sketch if you will.

Sunday August 4th, the day Milo made his entrance at 4:05 pm. I worked that day and I was told in morning report that I was the nurse that would admit the new diaphragmatic hernia, and mom had been laboring at the U of U for days. I waited and waited ALL DAY, but no baby came that shift. Looking back now, Milo wasn't quite ready to face all the hard work he would be required to do once he entered the world. He was safe and comfy and didn't want to budge. So, after almost 72 hours of labor, Milo was taken by C-section that evening. Milo was brought across the bridge from the University of Utah to Primary Children's Hospital to be placed on ECMO since Milo's lungs were so sick. ECMO in a nutshell is a treatment that uses a pump to circulate blood through an artificial lung back to that baby.

Bedspace 33 is where Milo began his fight.... His journey.... with his mom and dad right beside him every step of the way.

For Milo's first week of life, he was quite stable on ECMO. Shelly and Jason learned as much as they could. In fact, Jason could pretty much be the doctor. I remember my first time taking care of Milo I introduced myself to Jason and he immediately asked me what pulmonary hypertension was. When I started explaining, he pretty much took over and explained it hands down better than I was able to. I apparently passed the test cause Shelly and Jason asked me to be Milo's primary nurse the first day we met.

Milo's first hurdle was surgery to repair his diaphragm. He did surprisingly well. He did have to be somewhat of a contortionist to keep the ECMO circuit flowing well. He was in a permanent back bend which was painful to look at. Milo at times would start to squirm, cry and act uncomfortable and Shelly was there to hold his little hand. Her voice was magical. Sometimes we had to administer more pain medications and other times her calm presence was all Milo needed.

It hadn't even been a week, and Milo had swooned all the nurses. We all fell in love instantly. Becca said he opened his big brown eyes, and she was in love. He loved his breast milk swabs. I think between the ECMO nurse and the bedside nurse we would fight who got to give it to him, because he loved it so much. It was the one thing we could offer him to treat him like a new baby boy. Kristi would hold Milo's hand and when she would take her finger away, he would swing his arm around looking for her. She would reach back and grab his hand and hold it until he would fall back asleep. No matter how hard Kristi tried to reposition Milo he would always turn his head back to the left side. He always had his own plans. Jaime said, when Milo was upset, he would grab her hand so tight and one day she just stood there for at least 5 minutes because he wouldn't let go and she couldn't bear to take her finger away from him. Everyone that cared for Milo fell in love. But it wasn't just Milo we fell in love with, it was Jason and Shelly. There wasn't a day that they didn't thank the nurses for their service. There were always smiles when they walked into the room. Jason apologized constantly for his 100 questions. Which, I'm not going to lie, made me sweat. Although, I kinda liked it, because it kept me on my toes and I learned right along with them. They were the most gracious human beings. They always would ask us if we had gotten our lunch break. They would even sneak us in brownies, cookies and cakes from parent hour lunch. They took care of us, while we took care of their son.

On day of life 8, Milo started to have complications that were unclear to the medical team. Milo's liver was beginning to fail, his heart ultrasound showed worsening right heart pressures despite the interventions and a small left ventricle and aorta. It looked pretty grim, but I remember the day that the cardiac team came into the room to speak to Jason and Shelly and told them with the upmost confidence that they could fix Milo's heart if his lungs could be strong enough to come off ECMO. Shelly walked into that room with the biggest smile on her face. She said, "I can handle a long road, I just can't handle to hear this is the end". We were all hopeful that Milo could get off ECMO and his lungs could do his thing.

August 15th.... The day we challenged him to see if his lungs could support him off ECMO. Jason and Shelly were hopeful. We wanted Milo to soar, but we were scared it was not going to go well. Wow did he prove us wrong! We gave Milo a solid C on his hyperoxygenation test. It wasn't Milo's most shining moment, but we told Jason and Shelly that C's get degrees. We then trialed him off ECMO, and expected him to fail within a few minutes based on his C. We were shook (per Jen Mills) when he maintained his oxygen saturations for a good 15 minutes before they started to decline, and it took him 30 minutes before he showed us that he wasn't ready to come off. We gave him a B+ and a then we upped it to an A- to give him the benefit of the doubt!!! It was so exciting; we were all standing around just smiling and whispering to each other that we didn't expect him to do that well. At this point we knew Milo wanted to continue to fight and wasn't ready to gain his wings.

August 18th.... A small trial off was done and Milo didn't do as well. We talked with Shelly and Jason about new medications and treatments to help relax his pulmonary bed and relieve his pulmonary hypertension while improving his lung ventilation. Shelly and Jason made it clear that they didn't want to put Milo through any more pain and suffering, especially if the interventions wouldn't necessarily work or help him. They expressed concern about Milo's quality of life off ECMO. Would his little body make it to cardiac surgery? Could he tolerate other abdominal surgeries?

Shelly and Jason were realistic yet extremely hopeful. Every decision they made was out of love, never fear. Their decisions seemed to always be in sync with each other. They discussed hard things with such grace and poise. They trusted the medical team. They didn't want to be selfish and keep Milo here on this earth because they wanted him here. They wanted what was best for Milo. They wanted to make sure that they weren't the ones giving up on Milo. They wanted clarity knowing they did everything they could, and that Milo was going to be the one to tell them when he was tired and wanted to return home.

August 19th…. The medical did all the last ditch efforts in helping Milo's lungs open and ventilate. There were huge risks involved, yet Milo sailed through the procedure like nobody's business. The room went from being tense to some light laughter and cheering Milo on. (Shelly was doing the cheering, while Jason was asking all the questions…..like ALL the questions). Milo's lungs actually looked a bit better on xray.

Milo was then switched to our very strongest ventilator, to help gain more lung function. At this point Shelly and Jason knew if it didn't work, we were out of options. After 48 hours, Milo's pulmonary hypertension wasn't improving, and his liver was failing.

It was at this point that Shelly and Jason felt that Milo had done enough and was letting them know that his little body could no longer support him, and that it was time for him to return home.

Shelly and Jason held Milo all day long. We offered to take Milo outside, but Bedspace 33 became Milo's home, his sacred ground. Where his journey started and where Shelly and Jason wanted to end his journey. They held him, sang to him, told him stories, took pictures. We made a killer playlist for him.

We heard Jason whisper, "thank you for choosing us, thank you for allowing us to be your parents." Milo indulged one last time sucking up his mama's milk on a swab. We even indulged at the bedside with a cart full of contraband treats. We may have or may have not been in trouble, but I will never forget the smile on Jason's face when he found a fig bar in the treat stash. There was laughter, humor, tears and all the emotions. But Jason and Shelly knew they did everything. And Milo was ready.

<u>Milo gained his wings and left this earth gracefully and peacefully on August 23, 2019. Mighty Milo will be missed. Till we meet again.</u>

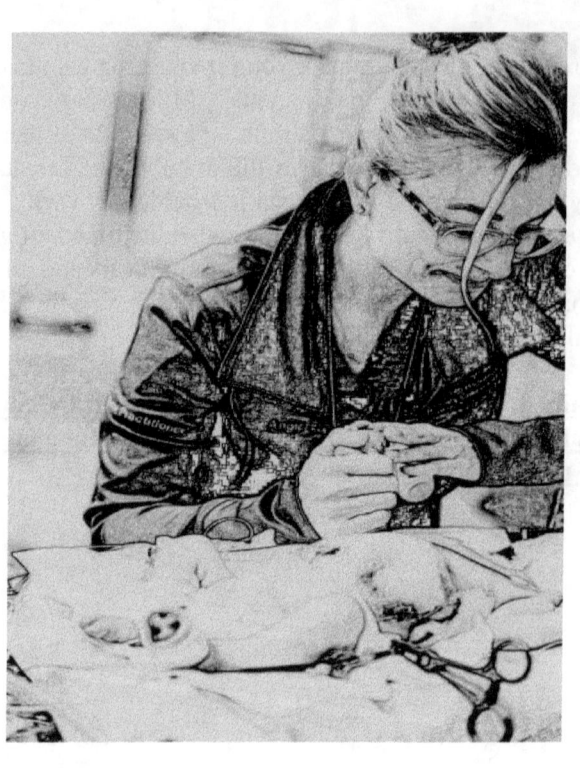

Letters to Milo Myers

Written by: Shelly Myers – my mommy

Shelly Myers

September 27, 2019 ·

Hi sweet boy,
We went to see you tonight. That makes two times this week - I know you loved all the visits. It's such a special place, that little grassy field filled with all you beautiful babies. I'm so grateful you're in such good company.
This week has been pretty good all things considered. But I've been missing you lately. Bad.
I need you to know that I know the end.
I know our family will be whole again in a day not far off.
I know you're always close - because I feel you.
I know you're ours forever, and that you're safely in the arms of our Savior.
I know this was your purpose and the way your life here was supposed to be.
But even knowing all of that doesn't make hard moments any less hard. It doesn't make this time without you pass any quicker. Knowing all of that doesn't fill my empty arms or heal the ache in my heart. It doesn't make each morning easier as your dad and I wake up and realize that we're still parents without our baby... that your crib is empty and your room is quiet.
Knowing everything I know helps me keep a view that's bigger than just right now, and it helps me feel hope and peace. I don't know what I would do without that, and I am very grateful.
But it doesn't mean I can't and won't cry at the hard parts. It doesn't mean I don't miss you, long for you and feel incomplete without you.
Please know that you're deeply missed, Milo. But more than that, please know that you're fiercely loved.
All my love,

Mom
#letterstomilo

Shelly Myers

October 11, 2019 ·

Hello beautiful boy,
A sweet friend brought by this card today. It's simple, but it articulates the feelings of my heart so well. You are such a light, Milo, even now. You have left a mark on this world, on so many hearts, on so many lives. You are truly mighty in every sense of the word. And I just want you to know how much I love you, how much I miss you, and how blessed I feel to be yours.
Your dad and I are sending up your 2 month birthday balloon today - forgive us for being late. But keep an eye out and tell the angels to grab it for you. It's a beautiful day without a cloud in the sky, so it should come right to you 😊
I love you, I love you, I love you.
Don't you ever forget it, sweetheart.
All my love,
Mom 🤍
#letterstomilo #mightymilo

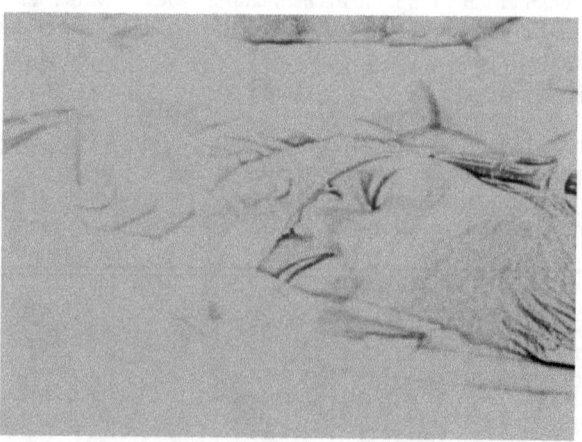

Shelly Myers
October 15 at 11:53 AM ·

There are things in life that just aren't fair. That are hard. That are heavy.

Losing a child is one of those things.

I've hesitated to write on a hard day because I don't want anyone thinking I don't love the life I have. I don't want anyone thinking I'm not grateful for the precious time I had with my son. And I don't want anyone sending me to the hospital because they think I don't want to live.

Let me be clear - I am grateful for every single day I have. Maybe now more than ever before. I love my husband and the beautiful life we've built. And I am deeply grateful for my son and the moments I had with him.

But I would be lying if I said I don't think about death often. I would be lying if I said I don't look forward to the day I get to hold my boy again. And I would be lying if I said that life doesn't look very different to me now than it used to.

When you lose someone you love, it completely shakes your world and your view of everything in it. Everything feels meaningless and trivial in comparison to the love and heartache that you simultaneously feel in every single moment after that person is gone. You are excruciatingly aware of their absence and all the things you're missing out on. In our case with Milo, every milestone he didn't experience, every smile we didn't see, and every sleepless night that would have been interrupted by him.

When you lose a child, you hate that you're able to sleep in because their nursery is silent. You hate that the carseat in the back is crumb-free and totally empty. You hate that you can't bring yourself to take that carseat out of the car because it's just one more thing separating you from them and parenthood. And you hate that you feel a twinge of sadness or anger or a million other feelings when you see other happy families going about their everyday lives.

You aren't angry with anyone else for having what they have - you're just angry that you don't have it too. But you aren't even really just angry. You're sad. And it's a sadness unlike anything you've ever experienced, and it often shows itself as anger. But when you sit down with it and really stare it in the face, you see that it's sadness... it's grief... it's love that's so big that it fills up your heart and comes out your eyes in big wet drops.

See, there's the before and the after. There's all the hopes and dreams and the life you always pictured before your person left... and then there's now. The reality, the things you've missed, the stark contrast of what you expected and what you have now that they're gone.

You find yourself placing so much value on the lasts - for us, it's the last moments in that sacred hospital room, the last time looking at Milo, the last seconds holding him, talking to him, and seeing him full of life. Those things become so etched in your memory and in your heart that they become untouchable and reverenced. And you ache for them to be real again.

There's also this insatiable desire to just feel normal. To be able to be happy doing everyday things, to be able to talk about your person without everyone feeling weird, to be able to make eye contact with your friends or family who have what you've lost and now feel guilty.

It's all such a hard, hard thing. It's a messy, raw and beautiful place to be. Because you are living everyone's worst nightmare, you can handle the hard and scary that anyone else wants to share with you. Because you've become friends with grief, it's freeing to talk about life's trials and have other people share with you. It makes it all feel meaningful knowing that you can be a shoulder, a rock or a listening ear for someone else as they navigate their difficult moments.

Losing Milo has wrecked me. I hate that I'm not home with him snuggling on the couch or walking to the park. I hate that I only have so many pictures to look at, and that he'll never be older than three weeks in my mind. I hate that my husband and I are parents without our baby.

But I am so grateful to have had him. I am grateful to have carried him safely with me for nine perfect months. I am grateful to have spent nineteen beautiful days with him. I am grateful that Jason and I are parents - that when someone new asks us if we have children, we can answer yes and tell them about our mighty boy. I am grateful for my family, my friends, my nurses and doctors who have all rallied around us and shown us that the core of humanity is so, so good. I am grateful for my husband who has never embodied the title of best friend more than he does right now. And I am grateful for a God who loves me and my Milo more than I can even comprehend - that He has my son safely in His arms, and that He is anxiously waiting for the day when He can place Milo back into mine.

Losing a person you love is hard. And it's totally okay to acknowledge that - to have horribly hard days and to be angry, sad and downright heartbroken. But losing someone you love also opens up your heart in a way nothing else can, allowing so much good, so much light, and so much love in.

#MightyMilo

Shelly Myers

October 28, 2019

Hello my beautiful boy.
Your stone was placed today and sweetheart, it looks so good. You'd totally love it. Your dad and I sure do.
Maybe it's because we know your cute face will make all the other moms and dads smile when they come visit their babies. Or maybe it's because it finally feels like you have a permanent spot that's all yours - like you've literally left a mark on the world. Or maybe it's because we get to see your handsome little self now every time we come visit. Whatever the reason, today felt so good. And visiting you just made us so happy 🤍
I know it isn't quite the family picture we wanted to be taking right now, but any picture with you fills our hearts. You fill our hearts.
Milo, you are so mighty. You bring unbelievable joy. And your life, your fight inspire so many. You are incredibly loved. Not just by us, but by countless others. I hope you can feel it every single minute of every day. We'll be back to visit soon, sweetheart.
All my love,
Mom 🤍
#letterstoMilo #MightyMilo

Shelly Myers is with Jason Myers and 6 others

December 2, 2019 ·

Hello love.
Today is the second day of December, and I wanted to write you a special kind of note. This month it seems like the whole world changes a bit - it takes more time to focus on the Savior, to serve one another, and to love a little more and a little better.
So I wanted to write you some special letters telling you about the people I treasure who have loved you, me, and your dad - and who have truly embodied the goodness of Christ.
Side note: I also thought it was pretty neat that I started writing this a few days ago before I found out that today's **#lighttheworld** challenge is to share about someone who gives Christlike service. So checking that one off.
Today's letter is about your incredible team of nurses and doctors at the hospital.
The NICU isn't really the first place most parents want to be with their new baby. It's foreign. It's sterile. It's full of machines and tubes and wires and lots of scary looking things. It's full of strangers. And if you're there, it usually means something is wrong.
But Milo, that place became your home. It became a hopeful, beautiful and peaceful place. Those machines kept you with us. Those strangers became our family. Our time there with you became sacred and holy. And so much of that was because of your team.
They loved you so much. They cheered you on every single day, every time you had a procedure, every moment you were with them. I watched how they cared for you. I saw how gentle they were - how they would hold your hands, brush your hair, and constantly make sure you were as comfortable as possible. They were the ones who spent the long nights with you. They were the ones who changed you, cleaned you, fed you and comforted you when I couldn't. They were the angels I prayed for.

Every day those beautiful men and women sacrificed time with their own families, their own babies, to take care of others. To take care of you. They are selfless. They are loving. They are Christlike.

I remember the way that

Jamie Cram York

was always so aware of the little things. She made sure your lips weren't chapped. She put lotion on your little hands and feet. She even washed and styled your hair after your first big procedure. She always cared for you the way a mom would - the way I would. I loved that about her.

I remember the way

Kris Christensen

would look at you. Her eyes would soften and sometimes she'd get this big, beautiful smile. She was so protective of you and made sure that your space was safe and that everything was working the way it should. I think she loved you a little bit extra because her family has a sweet IVF baby too, so she knew how much we wanted you and how hard we worked for you.

I remember the way

Avie Dougherty

fell for you. It was instant. She loved you the second she met you, and I always knew she would come in and visit you when I wasn't there. She's the one who made you your Mighty Milo sign above your bed. She was the first face I really remember from the NICU, and she always made me feel at home there. She loved you so quickly and so deeply. It makes my mom heart smile still.

I remember the way

Cindy Bond

smiled when she talked about you. She's been working with sick babies for decades, but she somehow keeps her big heart open and keeps loving the little ones she cares for. She even still cries when she loses a baby - she hasn't become calloused, and that is incredible.

I remember the way Dr. Chan worked so hard to think of every possible thing we could do to help you, to save you. She is smart and practical and was always there to help us think clearly and do what was best for you. She always had you in mind, and she always encouraged us to put your comfort and your quality of life first.

I remember the way

Lindsay Rees Nielson

cared for us. She would sit and talk with us late into the night while we were at your bedside. And she wrote me the sweetest card when she came to your memorial. She told me how much of an impact you had on

her and how you were one of the reasons she loves what she does... because she gets to take care of sweet little ones like you.
I remember the way
Jen Mills
sat in your room with us. She was always busy, but she pulled a computer in to the empty bed space by yours so she could stay close. She just sat and talked with us. She became our friend, and she always took the time to explain how things were looking and answered any questions we had.
I remember the way Sharon would talk with and comfort us while we made hard decisions about your care. She was always gentle. She was always supportive and encouraging. And she always empowered us to make the choices and decisions we felt were right for you. She really helped us feel like good parents, and that meant so much when the amount of parenting we could do felt incredibly limited.
I remember the way Dr. Yost would come over just to check on you. He is such a good man. And he's such a good doctor. He really cared about how you were doing. He must have been incredibly busy, but we'd see him pop into your room from time to time or after a big procedure to make sure you were okay.
I remember the way Dr. Yoder looked at your dad and I on your last day with us. His eyes were so sad. He was your very first doctor when you were born. He cared for you from day one when things looked so bleak. He watched your triumphs with a smile and always wanted the best for you. And he wished so badly for things to have gone differently. He was always so hopeful. I really loved that about him.
I remember the way
Rebecca Patton
cared about the little things. From giving you a pacifier to watching you gobble up milk, she was as happy as we were each and every time you were able to just be a baby. She wanted you to be nothing but comfortable on your last day. She worked hard to make sure everything was just right, down to the smallest detail. And as we got ready to turn off your ECMO machine, she sat with us and tried to help us be as ready as we could be. She gave you your final doses of medication to ensure you wouldn't feel any pain and that you'd go peacefully. In your final moments, she was there, still making sure that you were happy and that we were okay.
I remember the way
Angie Hall Birkeland
held you as she handed you over to us on our last special day together. She couldn't stop smiling. She couldn't stop talking about how

handsome you were. She was the one who helped dress you in your beautiful blue gown. She helped us create an unforgettable playlist for you - I can't listen to most of those songs without thinking about our last day together. She wanted everything to be absolutely perfect for us. She spoke at your memorial and helped everyone get to know your mighty little spirit. And she continues to reach out and remind me that it's okay to be sad, to be angry, to be happy and to be anything in between.

I remember the way
Kristi Kloepfer
cried for you. It both broke my heart and filled it to see the tears she shed for my son. She was one of the nurses who had the devastating job of caring for your little body after you left. I can't imagine what that must have been like. I apologized to her as we left the room that night because that just seems like the hardest thing in the world. But she said she was so grateful she got to be with you on your last day in the NICU as she was also with you on your first. She even came in early that night so she could be with us and be with you before we said goodbye.

I remember the reverence that Wendy had as she knelt in front of us and asked if we were ready to turn off ECMO. What a horribly difficult job. But she was graceful and kind. She had tears in her eyes and was so gentle with you. Your dad told me that he watched her and realized how beautiful the angel of death could be... that it wasn't scary like he'd always imagined. She made one of the hardest moments of my life holy. She is one of the sweet faces I see when I close my eyes and think of those last moments, and I am so grateful for the tenderness she showed us and you.

And I remember the way Ryann believed in you. You surprised her more than once with your fight and your mighty little spirit. I remember her telling the other doctors "you don't know Milo" when things looked bad and they didn't think you'd make it through a procedure. She clapped and smiled so big the first time they trialed you off ECMO. She was one of your biggest cheerleaders. She was also one of our biggest supports. She met with us before you were born and helped walk us through what we might face and work through tough decisions. And even now, she still reaches out regularly to see how we're doing. She remembers us. And she remembers you. And that means everything.

A lot of the members of your team came to celebrate your life at your memorial. It was touching and moving to see them there. Their hearts were just as involved in your daily care as their hands were.

Milo, these amazing people did absolutely everything they could for you. They did everything they could for us. I will never forget them or their kindness. I'll never forget the love I felt every day in that tiny hospital room. I'll never forget how incredible it felt to watch so many other people love my mighty son so deeply. To every one of your doctors, nurses, specialists and other staff members - thank you. You made all the difference. We love you very much.
All my love,
Mom 🤍
#letterstoMilo #lighttheworld

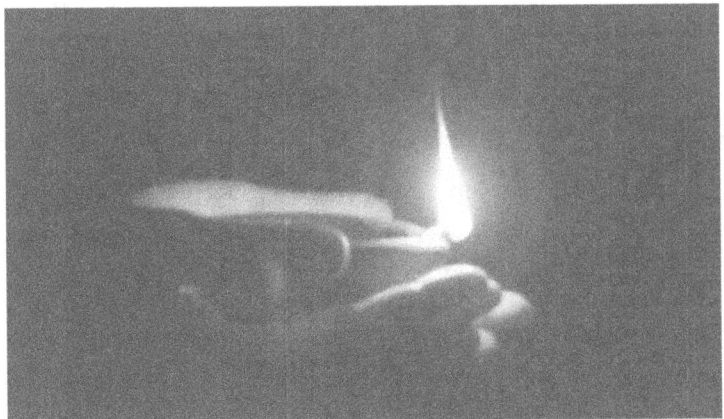

Shelly Myers is with Jason Myers.
December 16, 2019 ·
Hi beautiful boy.

Tonight I want to write you another special letter about someone we both love very much. He is one of your biggest fans and, lucky for me, one of mine too.

I want to tell you about your dad.

Now listen, I know that one letter will never do him justice. So just a heads up that there will be plenty more of these about that big guy we love so much.

I also know that you already know how incredible he is and how much he loves you. If there was an award for most involved parent in the NICU, your dad would have won. No contest. I remember how he would call the hospital every morning, right when he woke up. He'd usually get to talk to Avie, and he'd say that he was calling to see how his boy was - the Mighty Milo. He'd ask your nurses how you were doing. He knew every medication, every vital, every detail about your care. I think that was one of the things he felt like he could do to protect you and be there for you. And sweetheart, he was so good at it.

Your dad couldn't wait to meet you when you first came. He knew that our time with you was precious and that it might be brief. So as soon as he made sure I would be okay, he ran in to be with you. It was just the two of you for about a half hour. The pictures from that time are so precious to me. Photos of my husband with our son - it's something I had waited so long to see.

Milo, you mean the world to him.
You're his boy.

I know that if faith and courage would've kept you here, your dad could have done it single handedly. He believed in you. And he cheered you on every second he was with you in that little room. I remember him reading to you at night. After we'd finish "Mustache Baby" or "Leo the Lovable Lion", he'd pull out the scriptures and find stories of valiant, brave men who trusted in God and defeated adversity. He'd read to you about Daniel. He'd read to you about David. And he'd tell you that you were just as mighty. That you were just as strong. And that if God willed it, you could overcome anything.

He was right.
(Don't tell him, but he's right a lot of the time.)

You were able to overcome so much in your short life. Because you are mighty. Because you are strong. Because you are your dad's son. And because God mercifully let you stay with us for so much longer than we expected.

Milo, your dad is so proud of you. He loves you more than anything in this world - maybe even more than me. (How about we can just tie for first place though.) He loves to talk about you. He loves to look at pictures and videos of you. And when he meets someone new and they ask him if he has any children, he smiles and proudly tells them about his perfect son.

I wish you could see just how much he misses you. I mean, I know you can. Maybe even better than I can. In his quiet moments alone. When he cries. When he says your name. When he just can't be strong for one more second. The other night he said how he just wanted you here - how he just wanted to hold you. I wished more than anything that I could give him that. That I could give him you.

I know he's strong for me a lot of the time. But I know he has his hard moments too. I do my best to be there for him. To hold him. To just sit in the sad together. But maybe you could help me out, babe? I know you're busy working miracles with Jesus, but if you get a chance, could you come visit your dad for a little while? He'd love to sit with you, to be with you.

Milo, we're pretty lucky, you and me.
We somehow convinced God to give us your dad.
And he's the best person I know.

He prays for you every single night. He kisses your sweet little picture every time we visit the cemetery. And he still wears his hospital bracelet from the day you were born. He's never taken it off. Trust me when I say that you are never far from his thoughts or his heart. He loves you with everything he has, and so do I. I'll give him a big bear hug for you tonight.

All my love,
Mom 🖤

#letterstoMilo

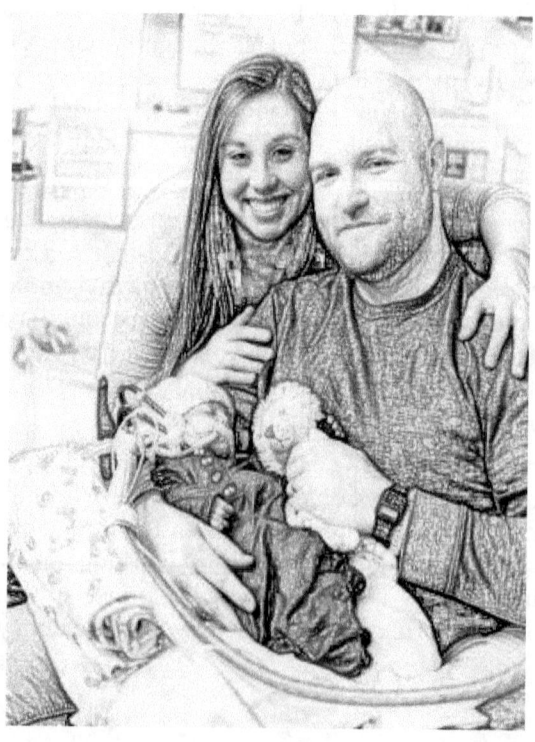

Shelly Myers

March 28 ·

I miss you x 1,000,000.
#letterstoMilo #MightyMilo

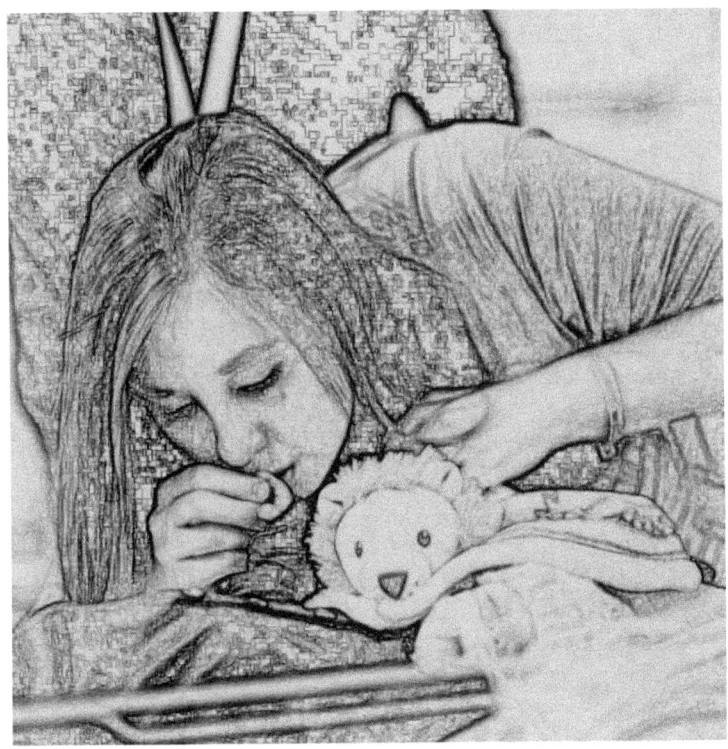

Shelly Myers is at Intermountain Primary Children's Hospital

June 4 at 12:22 AM ·

I looked at pictures and watched videos of you tonight and just cried. I can't explain how much I miss you. I can't describe the ache. It's always there, but some days (and nights) it's just more intense, more painful, more raw. It almost feels like I'm right back where I started... like I just lost you. It's all the same pain and heartache but without the comfort, without the divine strength and concourses of angels I know were near, without all the flowers and cards and hugs.

I can see a picture of you and instantly be right back in that NICU, holding your hand, watching your beautiful eyes find mine, grateful for every moment but also pleading with God to save you. I'm there. In an instant. I just wish you were there with me.

Today is your 10 month birthday. Your dad has always loved this age and has literally dreamt of the day that he'd have a baby this old. To play with and love on. It breaks my heart to know he doesn't get to have you here with him.

Milo, I'm scared to live a lifetime without you. I'm scared to lose you anymore than I already have. I'm scared to forget. I'm scared to make memories that you aren't in. I'm scared to move forward when you aren't physically here to do it with me. I'm scared to put a picture on the wall that you aren't in. I'm scared to be pregnant again because though it will be beautiful and exciting, it will also be complicated and hard and a constant reminder that you should be here as a big brother. Tonight I am so scared, so sad, and so broken. It comes and goes in waves, even nine months later. I hope you always know how much I love and miss you, Milo. You'll always be my boy.

All my love,
Mom 🩶
#letterstoMilo #MightyMilo

Shelly Myers

<u>April 2</u> ·

It's 1 am, and you are all I can think about.
The world is a little bit broken and in chaos right now, and so many people are afraid of what tomorrow brings. I feel for them because my world has been broken for months... chaotic in its own way because grief is unmanageable and completely unpredictable. And my tomorrows are a mixed bag because they're one day closer to you but also one day further from the last time we were together.
I miss you, Milo. Sometimes it's so much that it feels like a physical weight on my chest. I can't breathe. And I just wish you were here.
Just when parts of my heart feel like they may be healing, I see a new picture of you... a new video of you. I walk by your room. I see a beautiful newborn baby. I see your blanket. I hear one of the songs we played for you.
Milo, you are everywhere.
And I love that. So much. Because I need you everywhere.
But some days it also just breaks me wide open all over again. Because I can feel you so close, but you're still just out of reach. I can't hold you. I can't kiss you. I can't look into your eyes or see you smile. But by golly I feel you, and I'm so grateful for that.
Shakespeare said, 'Grief makes one hour ten.'
I think using that same scope, it has made these 7 months an eternity.
I love you, sweetheart. I miss you. And I can't wait until you're in my arms again. Send us some of that heavenly peace and divine comfort, okay babe? I think the whole world could use it.
All my love,
Mom 🤍
#letterstoMilo #MightyMilo

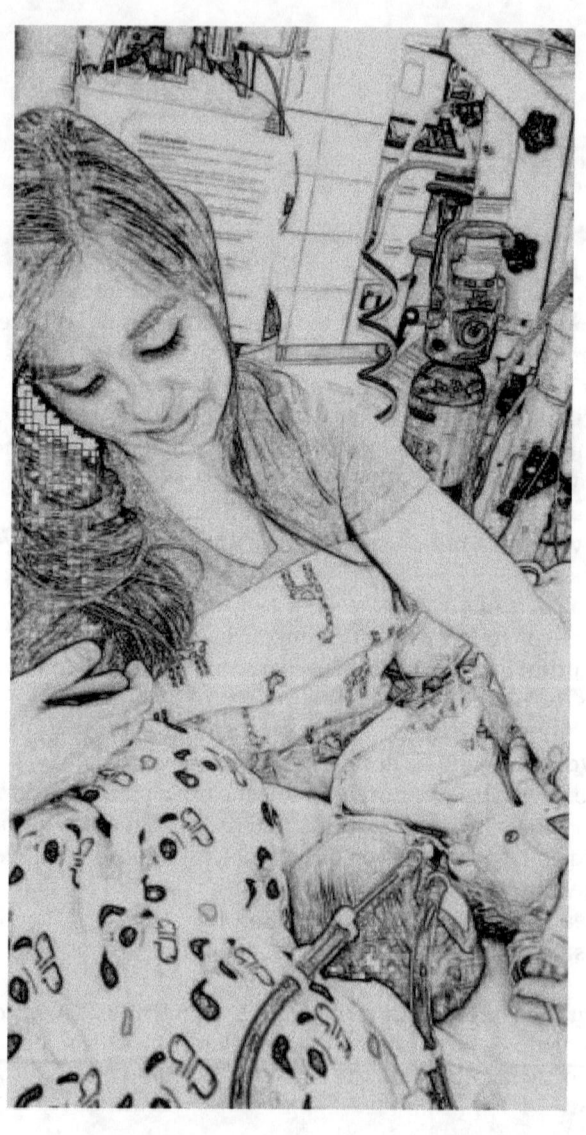

Shelly Myers

June 1 at 7:46 PM ·

Some days I just miss you extra.

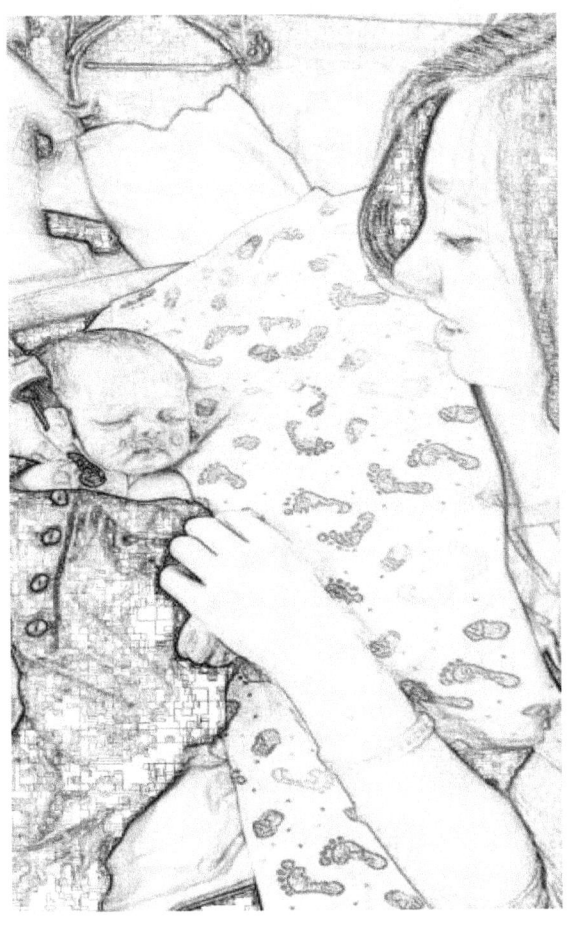

Hey mommy, it's Milo –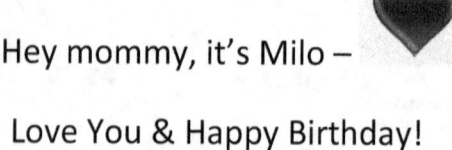

I Love You & Happy Birthday!

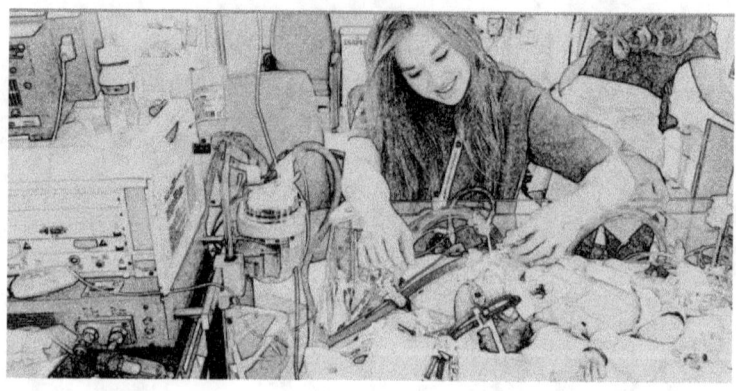

And tell daddy I love him too, he's my Hero!

Memories in pictures

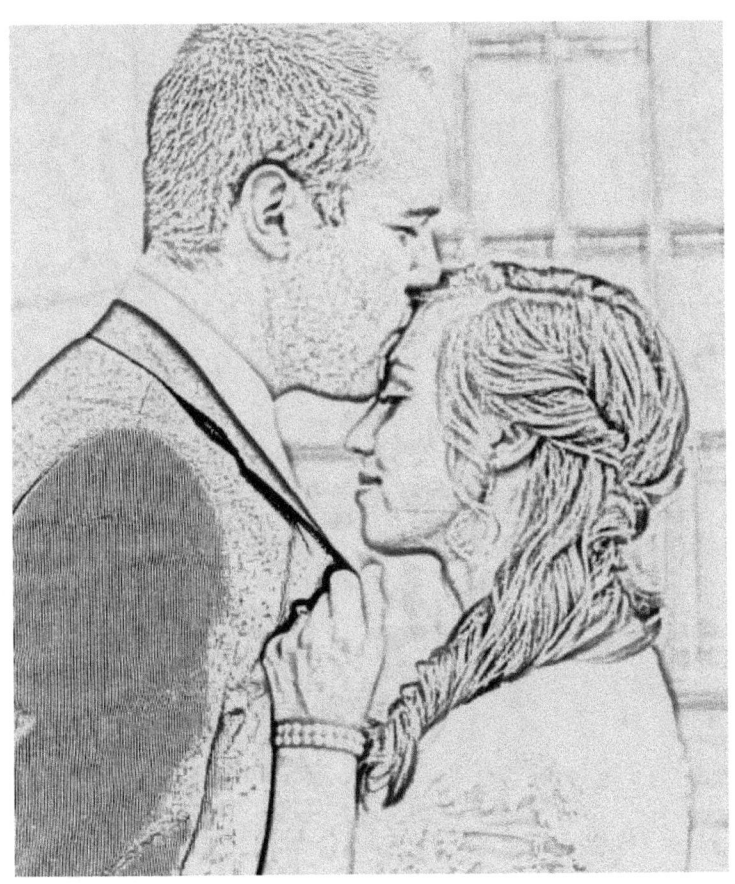

A very happy day!

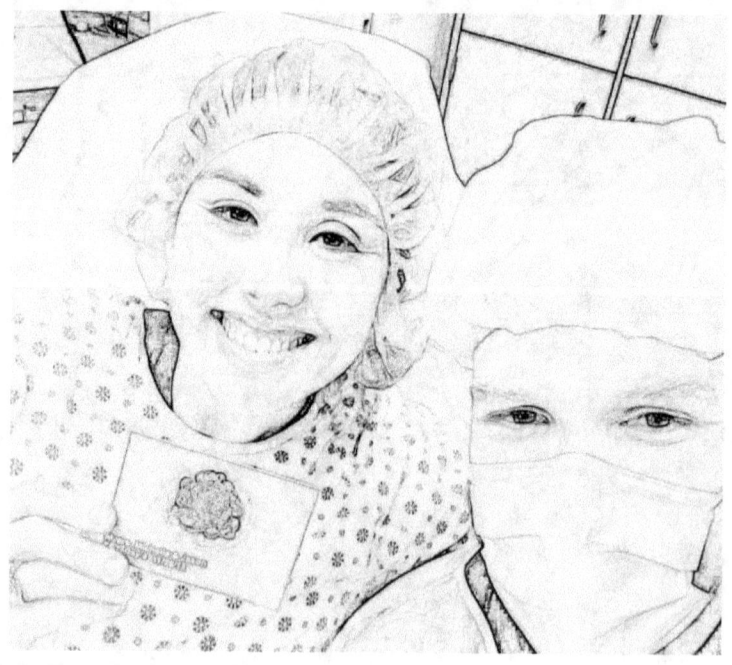

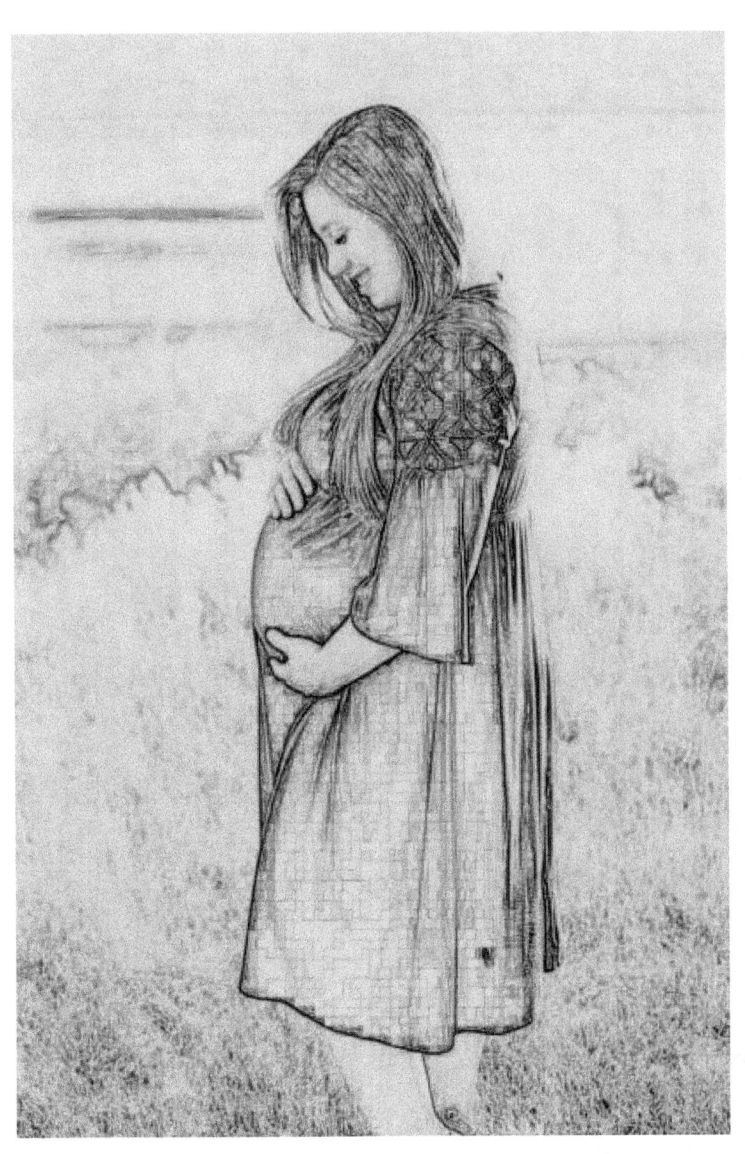

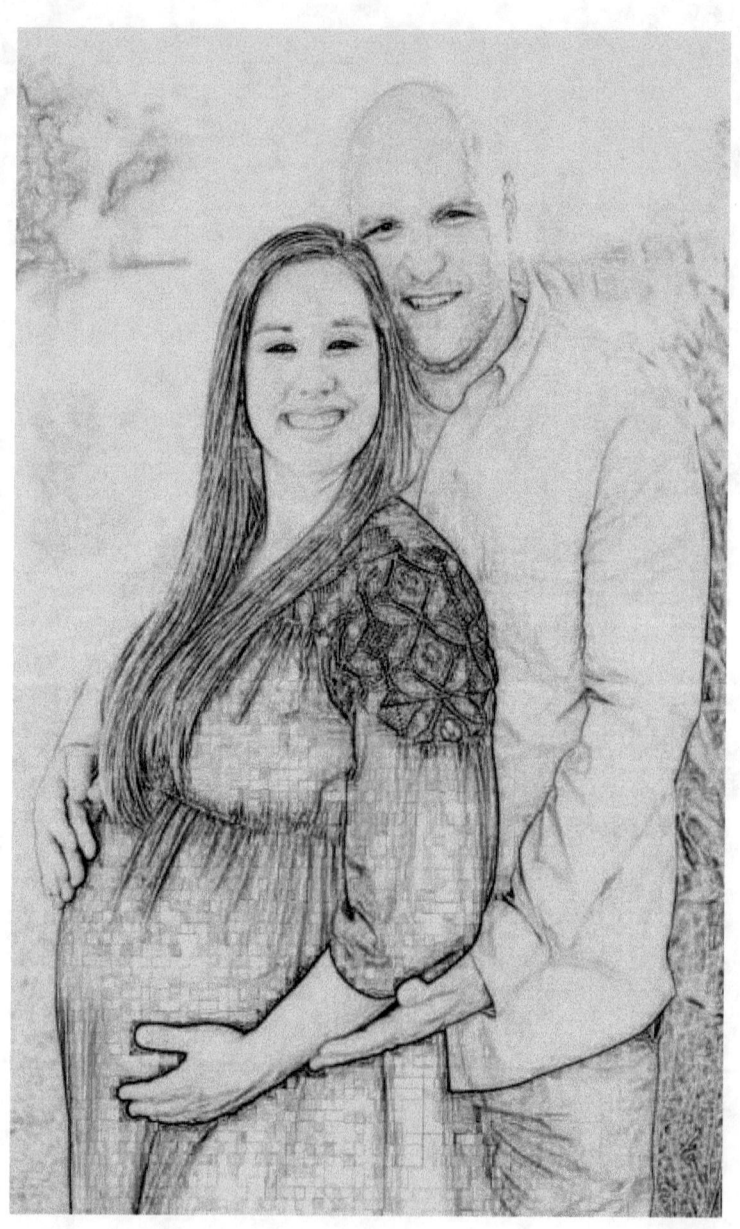

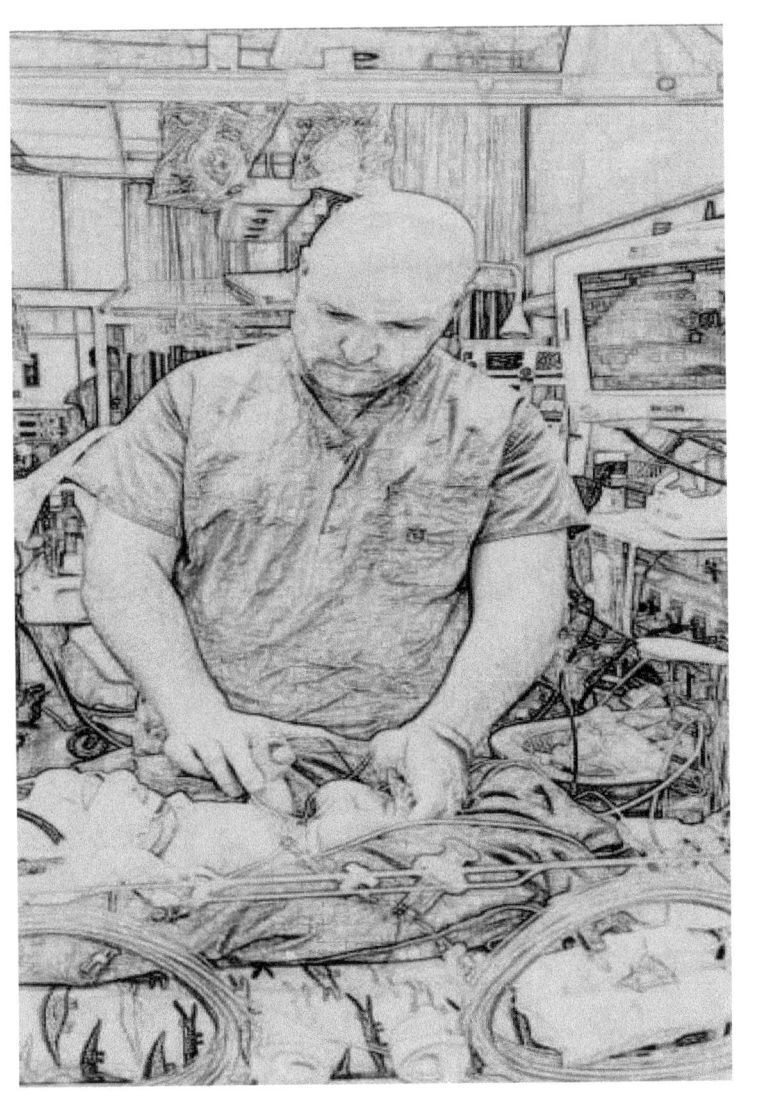

That tickles mommy...

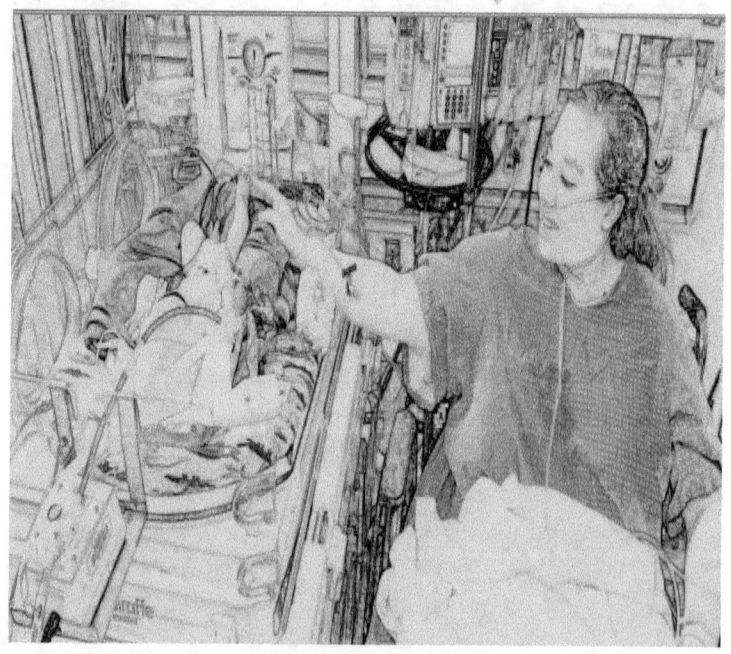

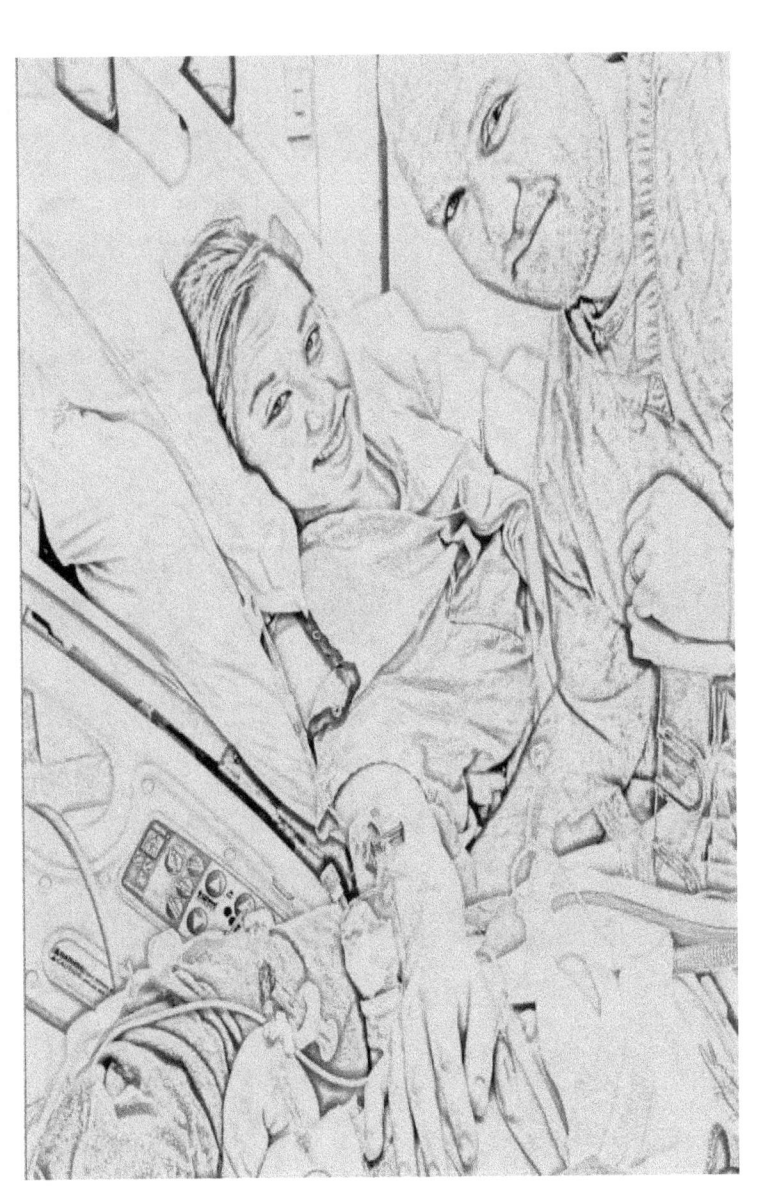

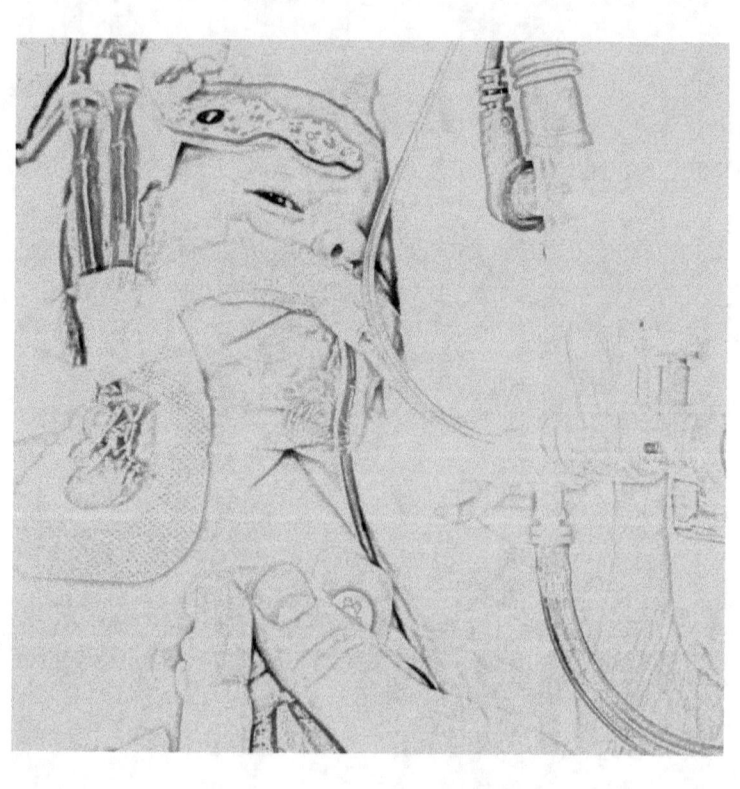

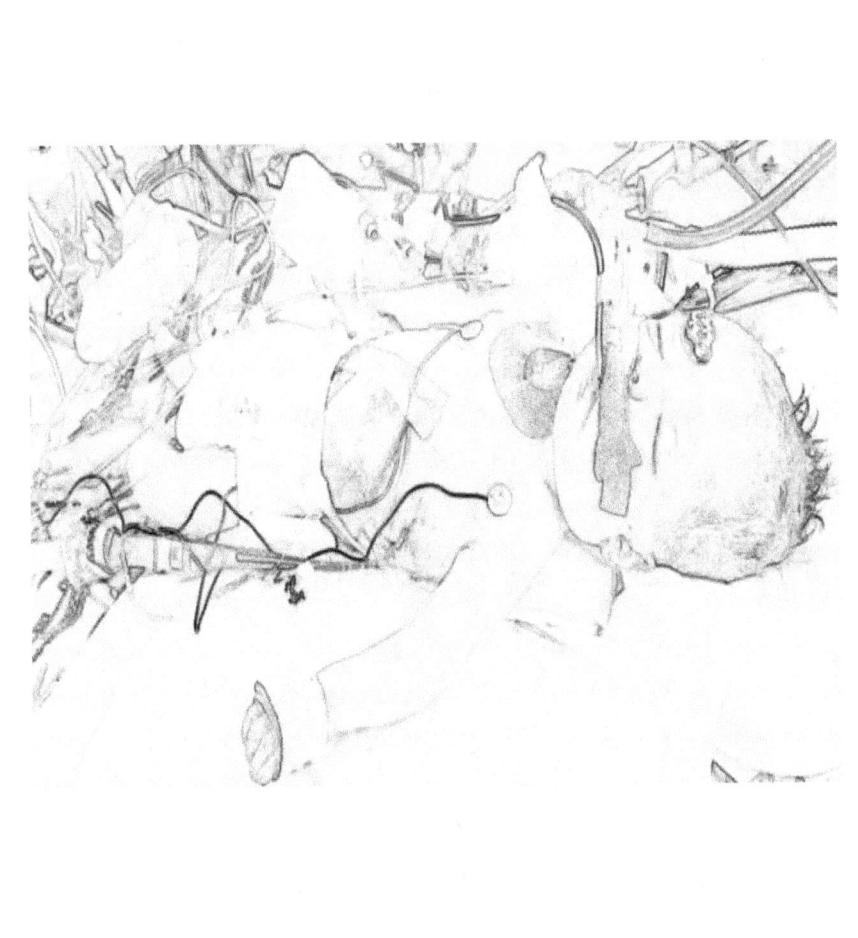

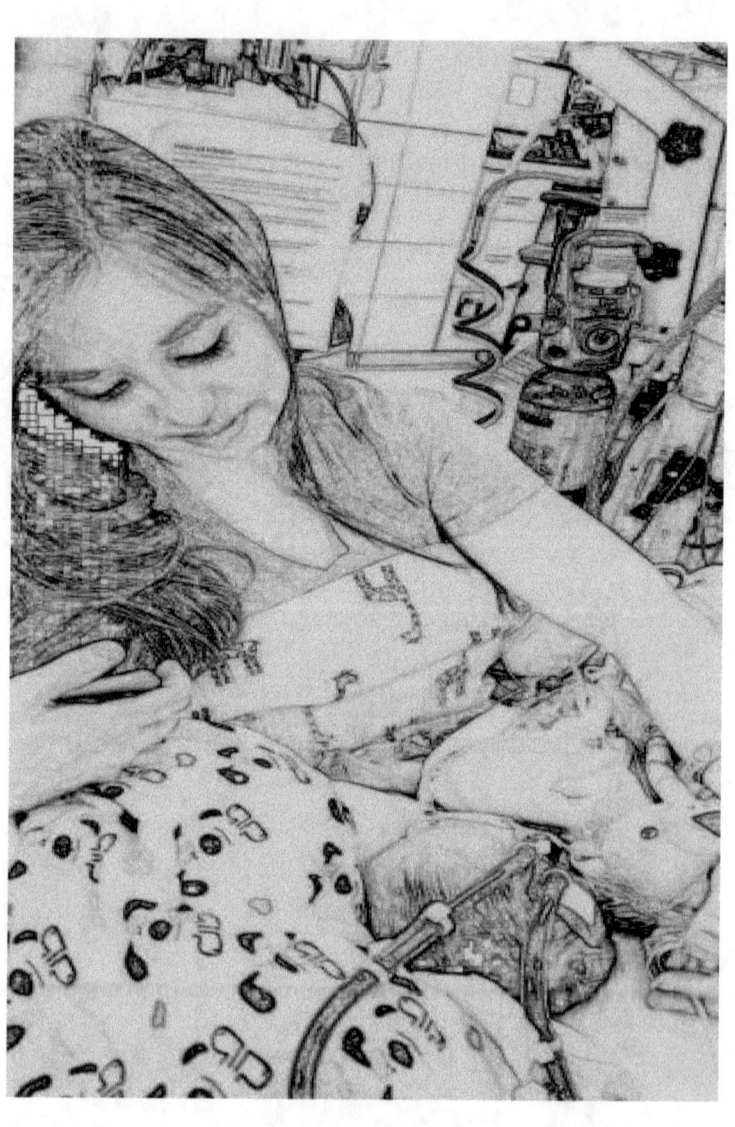

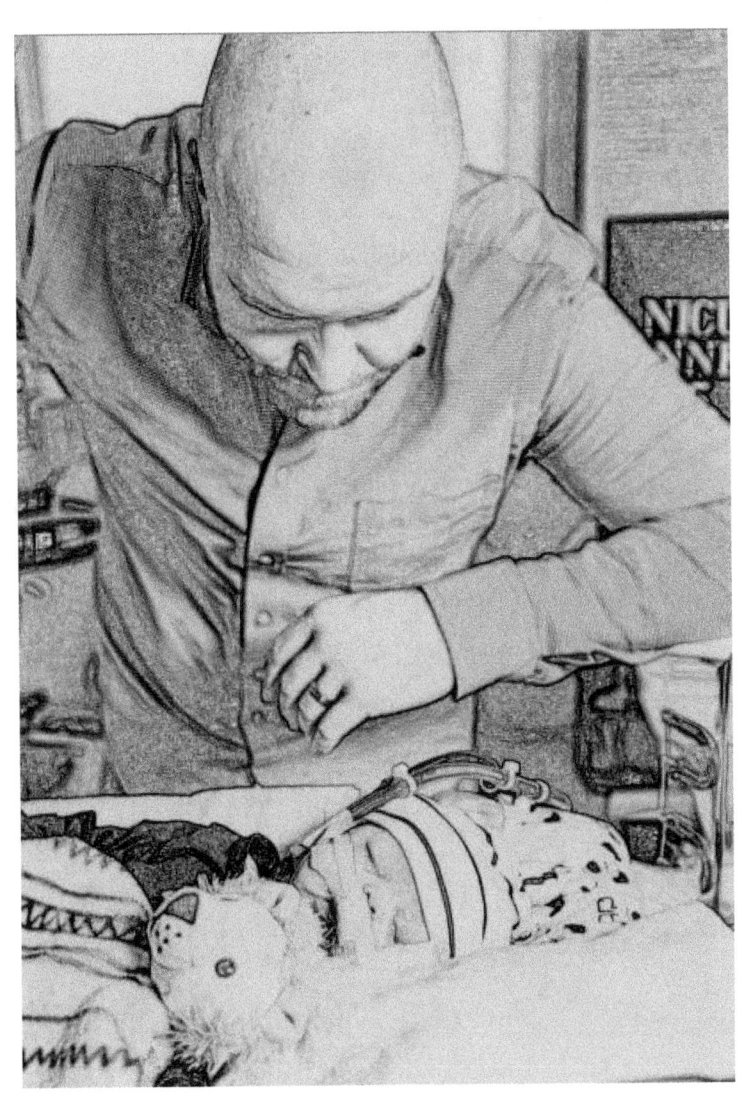

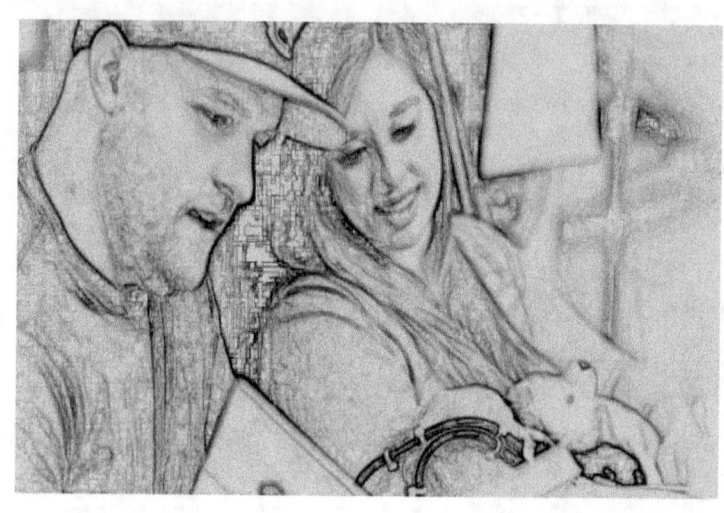

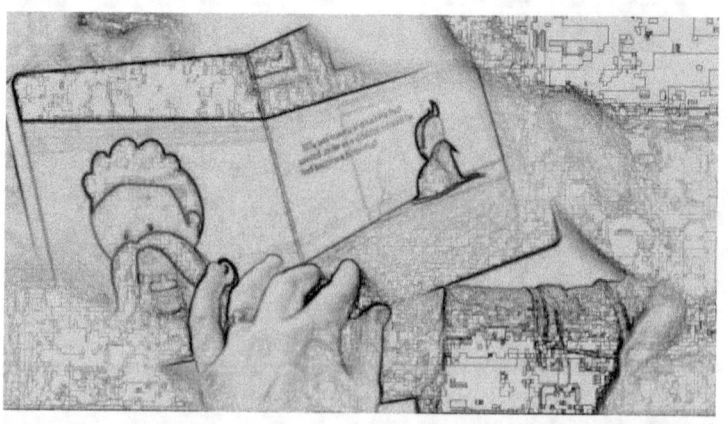

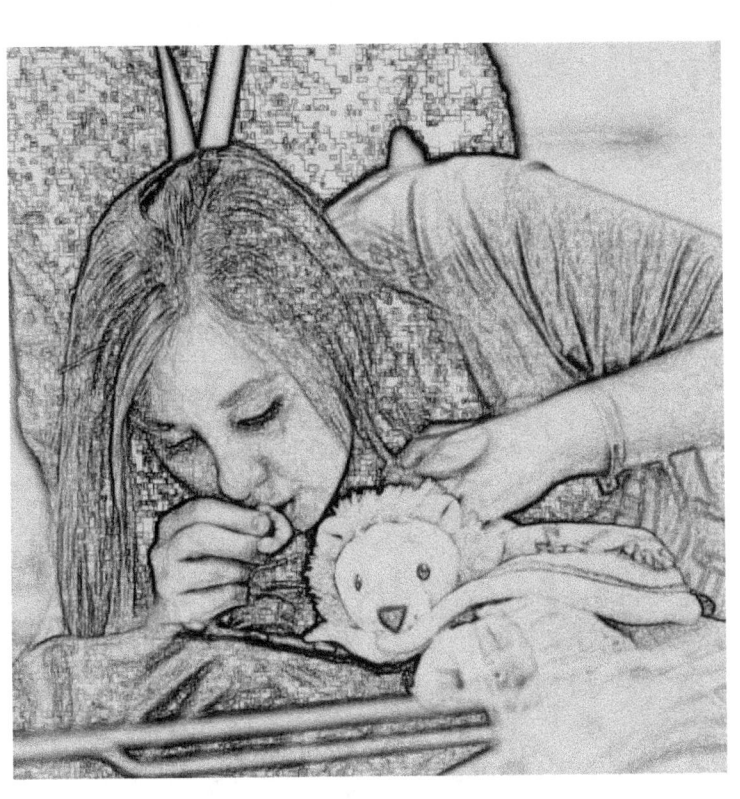

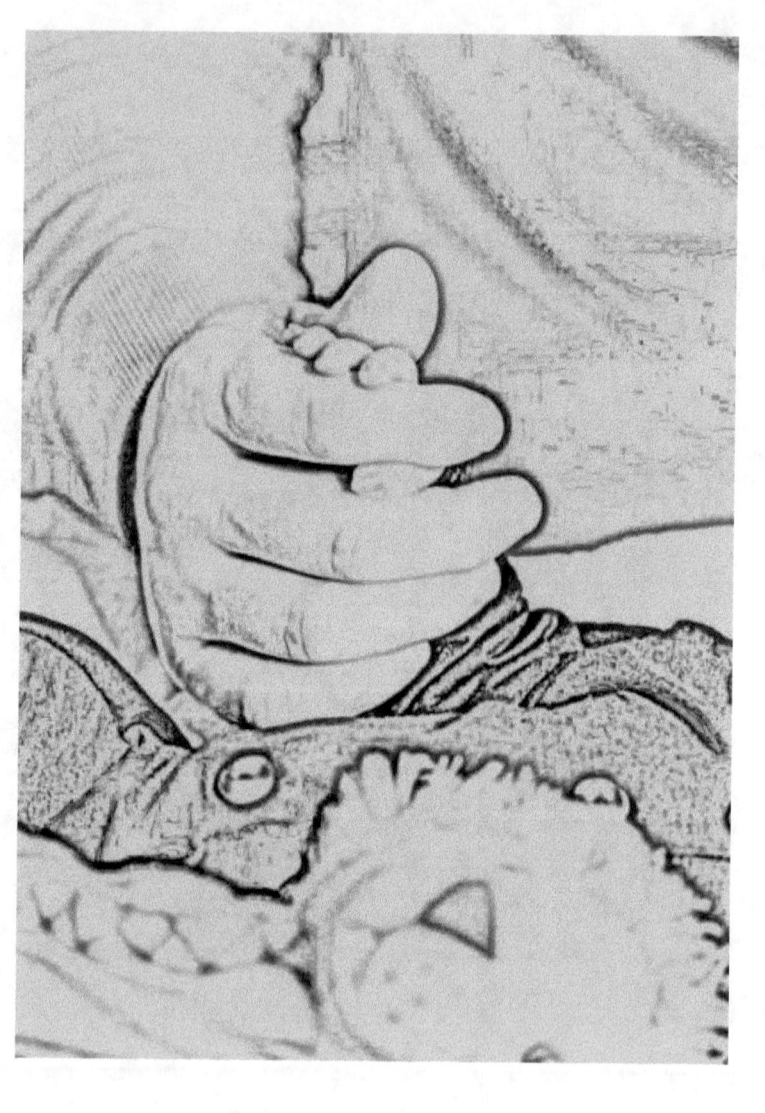

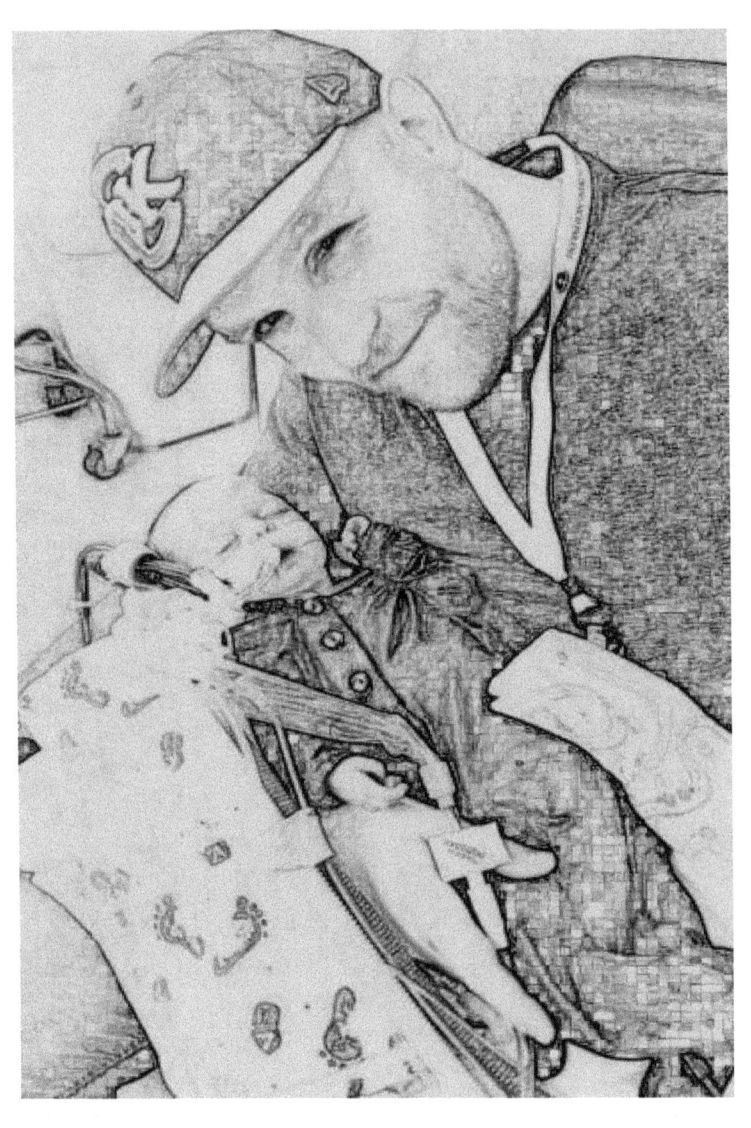

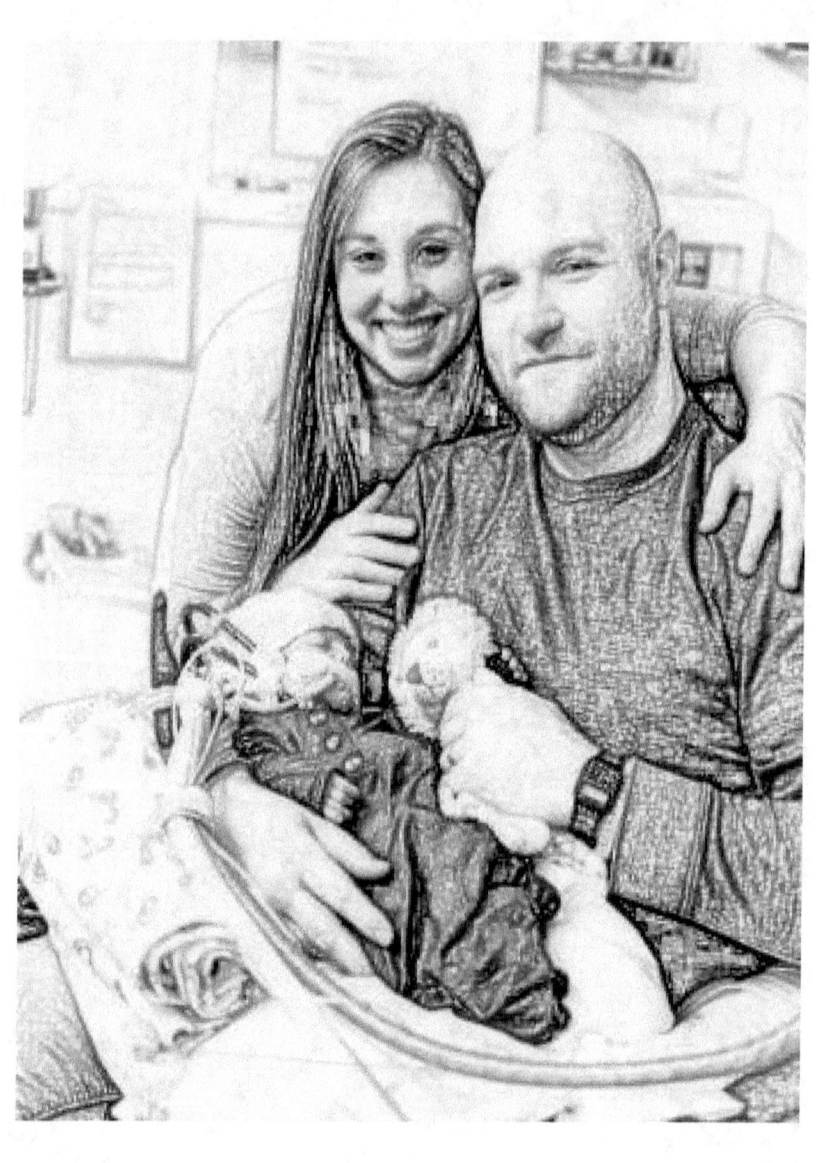

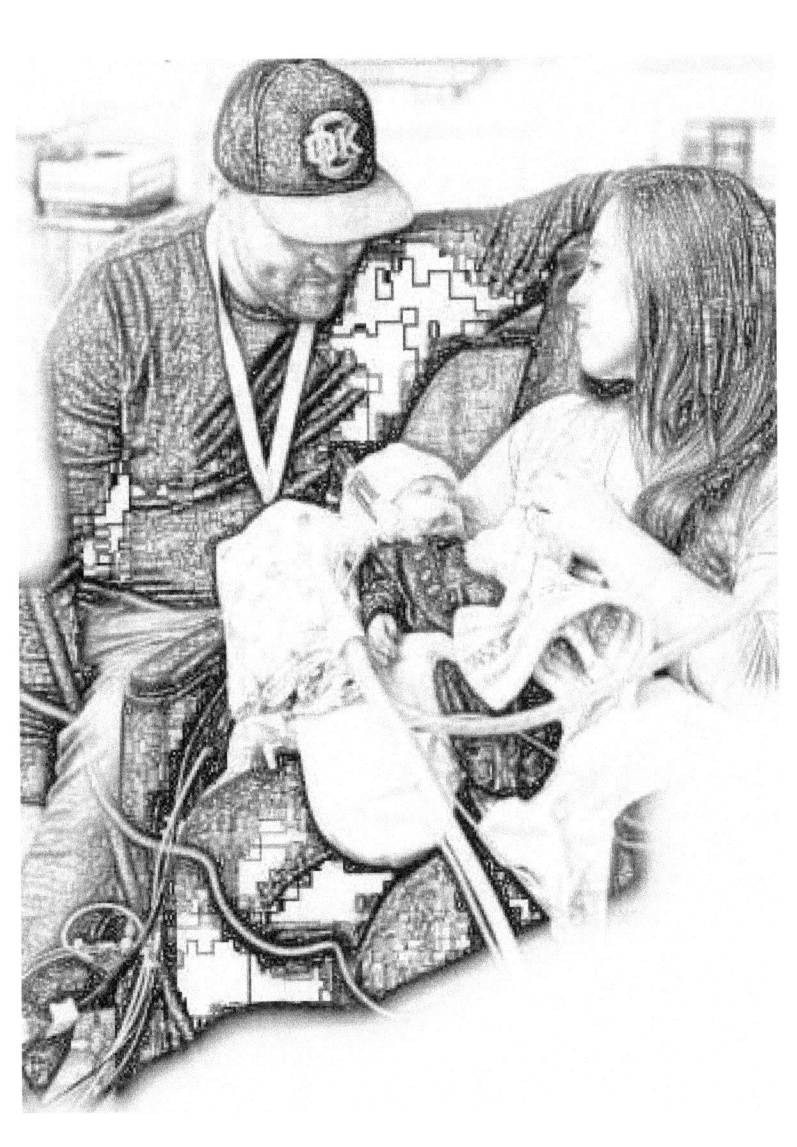

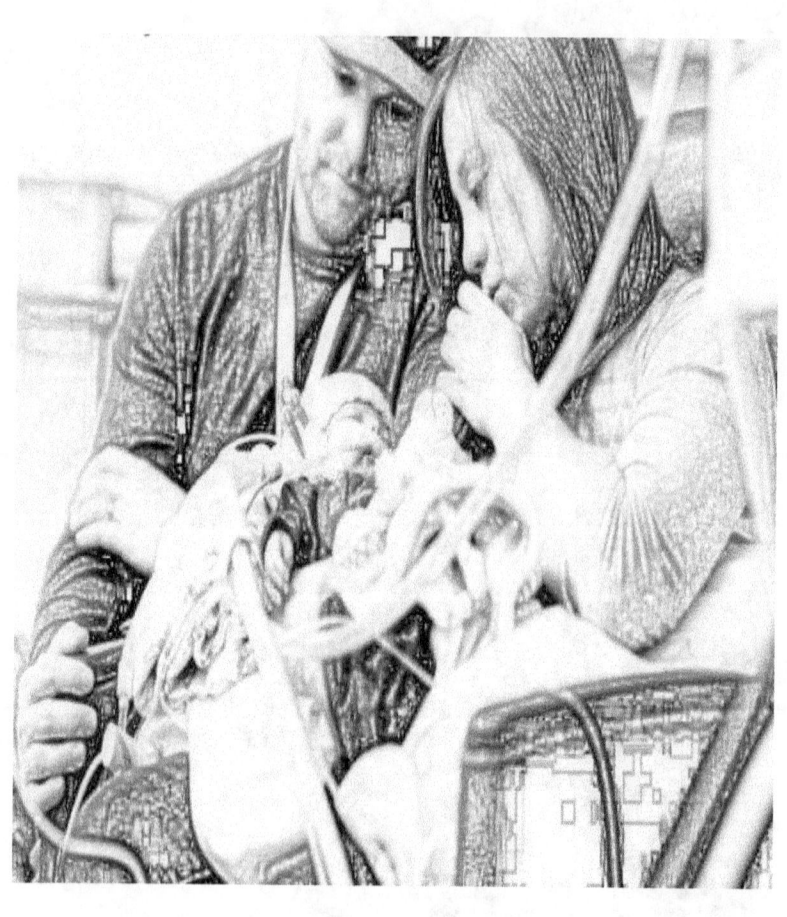

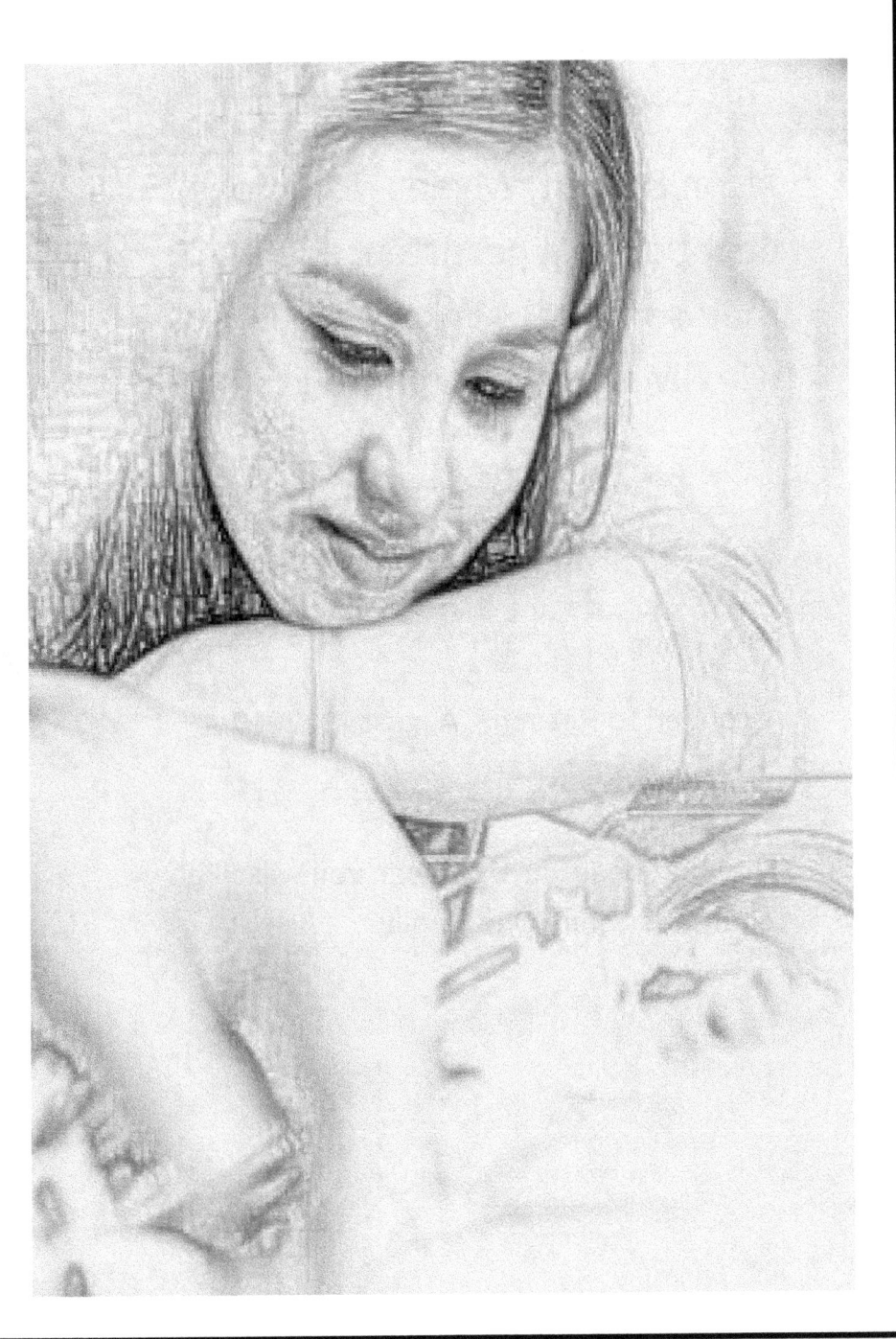

This book is dedicated to

Jason & Shelly Myers. Their love, devotion and persistence to help their son (Me) Mighty Milo Myers who lives on and on unto Eternity!

Mighty Milo Myers

Born – August 7, 2019

Ascended to Heaven – August 23, 2019

Until that beautiful day when you will all be together as one. One Family!

By: Nana Barby

www.ingramcontent.com/pod-product-compliance
Lightning Source LLC
Chambersburg PA
CBHW050259220526
45465CB00002B/751